Essential Oils:
25 Legendary Essential Oils Recipes For Quick Pain Relief

Table of content

Introduction

You have probably come across essential oils in many different areas of your life. Although the first thought to cross your mind may be oils being used for massage there are many potential ways to use these essential aromatic oils. An essential oil is simply an oily liquid which is obtained from almost every living thing. You will have smelt roses in the past or even a curry plant. The aroma is produced by the essential oil in the plant and there are a variety of methods of releasing this.

However, what you may not know is that an essential oil is considered to be a volatile compound! This is something that will quickly shift from one state to another under the right conditions. For aromatic oils the only condition required is temperature. The warmth of an average room is enough to convert the oil from a liquid state into a gas; this is the reason why you get an instant, almost overpowering aroma when you open an essential oil bottle. In gas form the essential oil can quickly move across a room and leave a delicate, yet beautifully balance aroma behind.

But essential oils are more than just a pleasant smell. For many years people have been using them to treat a variety of conditions. These can range from simple smelling salts to pain relief. It is currently believed that the oldest use of plants and their essential oils to treat a variety of issues can be traced to 18,000 BC. Cave drawings of this period in the Dordogne area of France show local plants being used to heal. Of course, Ancient Egypt is often associated with essential oils and the power of healing; their most famous mixture had at least sixteen different oils in and was perfectly adapted to being incense, perfume or even medicine! In the times of Ancient Egypt you needed to be a priest in order to use an essential oil; they were believed to be an essential part of coming close or even becoming one with the Gods.

Every single essential oil has its own distinct smell and can be used to help the body heal. However, you will also find that the right combination of oils can create medicine which is at least as powerful as the modern, man-made drugs so frequently prescribed today. All over the world these powerful essential oils are being used to help heal and provide pain relief to those who need it.

This book will provide you with 25 recipes to give you the right pain relief for any condition no matter where you find yourself. Some of these can be prepared and kept until needed but, in general, they work best when freshly made. It is worth noting that the quality of the essential oil occurring naturally in a plant can vary as the seasons change and even with the quality of the soil. If you intend to harvest these oils yourself it is best to ensure they have been grown in the best possible conditions.

Chapter 1 – 9 Simple But Effective Pain Relief Recipes

Pain is a fact of life that you will need to deal with at some point. It may be a short blast and quickly pass. However, at some point you are likely to find yourself in a more severe state of pain and wishing you had a cure for it. This is especially true if you start needing to take large quantities of pain medication. You can potentially become addicted or dependent upon the pain relief. A natural alternative does not offer this option; it simply provides pain relief. The following recipes will help you to deal with any pain issue:

1. The Muscle Ache

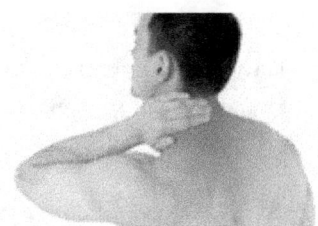

http://www.thephysicaltherapyadvisor.com/wp-content/uploads/2015/04/YoungManExperiencingNeckPain.jpg

This is something everyone will suffer with at some point, especially if you start exercising again after a short or long break.

Mix two drops of essential Lavender oil with four teaspoons of massage oil. Once you have combined them thoroughly you can massage some, or even all of the mixture onto the affected area. It will take a few moments to soak into your skin and will then work, directly on your aching muscles. You may be surprised at how quickly it can relax them and help you to feel better!

2. The Headache

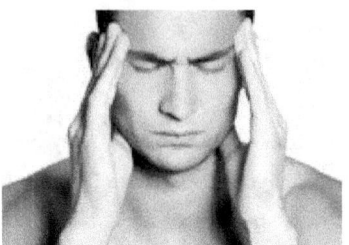

http://owwmedia.com/wp-content/uploads/Headache1.jpg

This is another lavender based recipe. This time, your two drops of lavender oil only need to be combined with a small amount of massage oil; such as half a teaspoon. The mixture will effectively be stronger and should work even more quickly although it should be used with caution.

To obtain pain relief simply apply the mixture to your temples and gently massage it in to place. Within a few moments you should feel warmth around the area and the pain will start to fade. Lavender has a fairly powerful aroma; if you are not happy with the smell it is possible to reduce it by adding a drop of another essential oil. However, it is important to choose the right one which will complement the pain relief process.

3. Menstrual Pain

This can be a particular difficult period for many women. It can often feel like the world is about to collapse around you. There is little which conventional doctors can offer except for the traditional pain relief approach. Fortunately, the following recipe will dramatically reduce or may even eliminate the pain and cramps:

You will need to mix together in a small bowl, fifteen drops of peppermint oil, five drops of lavender and ten drops of Cypress essential oil. Alongside this you will need what is referred to as a carrier oil; this is the base oil into which the essential oil is mixed. Sweet almond oil is a very popular choice when mixing essential oils.

Add two teaspoons to your mixture and stir thoroughly. You can then apply it gently to your stomach using a cotton pad and light, circular motions. It will take a few minutes to take effect.

4.Alternative Muscle Ache Remedy

This is an excellent recipe to alleviate the initial ache of your muscles after you have completely an exercise routine or when you first feel them straining. It requires you to mix sixty drops of Grapeseed oil with twenty of Jasmine. You can then add a few drops of Ylang Ylang. Once mixed you can pour this into a hot bath and climb in! It is best to soak for at least fifteen minutes to ensure your aching muscles have time to absorb the solution. It will relax them and you will feel much better when you climb back out of the bath.

1. Sore Muscles

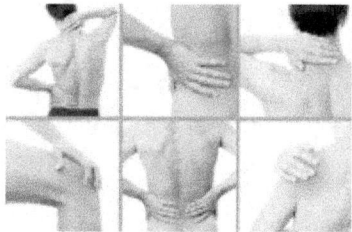

http://lethow.com/wb-content/uploads/2014/10/How-to-Treat-Sore-Muscles-Fast-and-Feel-Good.jpg

There is a difference between muscles which ache from general exercise and those which are in pain due to excessive use. Excessive exercise can create sore muscles; in turn this can make it difficult to move or even continue your exercise. In addition you may find sore muscles are exceptionally painful. Fortunately these can be generally avoided by applying the following mixture to them before you undertake any exercise:

Two drops of lavender oil can be mixed with the same amount of Eucalyptus oil. You will then need to add your base oil; again sweet almond is a good option. You will need eight tablespoons of this. The mixture created does not need to be used in one go; you can save some of it for future use. Massage the mix into your muscles before you start exercising and you will be surprised how much better your muscles respond.

If you have developed sore muscles from doing too much of any type of exercise then a mixture of three drops of Rosemary and three drops of Lavender can be combined with five teaspoons of almond oil. Again it will need to be massaged into the sore muscle; it is best to do this gently!

2. **After Exercise Aches**

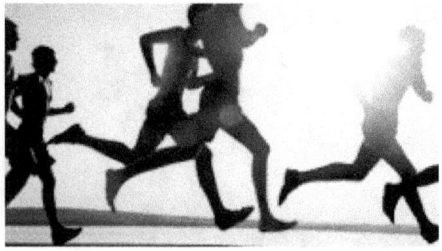

http://simpleeconomist.com/wp-content/uploads/2013/07/run.jpg

Undertaking exercise is good for your health; that is the official line! However, once the endorphins have finished making you feel good you will start to be aware of just how much your body is aching. Specific muscles will probably feel the pain more than others; depending upon the exercise you have undertaken.

To combat this it is advisable to mix four drops of Lavender oil with four drops of Juniper. You can then add six drops of Rosemary. Once you have mixed this thoroughly, you will need to add eight teaspoons of your base oil. You can choose any oil, although sweet almond is an exceptionally versatile and affordable option. Once you have mixed this simply massage it gently into the affected muscle. It is even effective if you have sore joints.

3. All Over Ache

You may find that you simply ache all over your body; there are a variety of reasons why this may be the case. This recipe is effective at reducing the pain associated with these aches. It is also effective at dealing with joint pain.

You will need six drops of Peppermint essential oil, five drops of Oregano and three drops of both Lavender and Cedarwood. Once you have mixed these oils together thoroughly you can add one and a half tablespoons of almond oil; this is the base or carrier oil. It can then be massaged directly onto the skin where you are experiencing the aches.

Aching all over can also lead to inflammation as your muscles and joints have been overworked. Your body will naturally compensate for any injured muscle; this can place a strain on other parts of your body and cause the inflammation. The following oils can be used to create an anti-inflammatory mixture which can offer effective relief: six drops of Chamomile oil, six of Lavender and ten of Frankincense. Finally add one two tablespoons of your base oil, ideally sweet almond. Then simply gently massage it into the affected area for inflammation relief. You can do this several times a day.

4. Sciatica relief

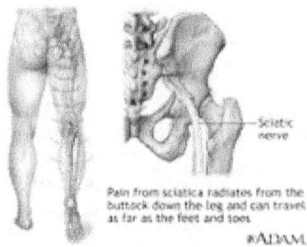

Pain from sciatica radiates from the
buttock down the leg and can travel
as far as the feet and toes

Sciatic
nerve

ªADAM

Sciatica is an extremely painful lower back pain which radiates down at least one of your legs and sometimes both. It can be deliberating as well as extremely painful! Fortunately it is possible to get some relief by mixing a few essential oils together and applying the mixture to the affected area regularly. Sciatic pain is often cause by a problem with the discs in the lower part of your back. Whilst the essential oils cannot help to fix this they can provide relief from the pain which accompanies this condition.

Mix four tablespoons of St. John's Wort oil with two tablespoons of olive oil and ten drops of geranium oil. You will then need to add six drops of peppermint and twenty drops of lavender. The mixture should be mixed thoroughly and then placed in a dark glass bottle and left in a cool place for twenty four hours. It will then be ready to use and you can apply it to the painful areas after a warm bath or a shower. The warmth of your skin will help it soak in.

5. General Pain relief

There are times when you simply need a concoction to hand which will work to reduce any painful part of your body in the minimal amount of time possible. The following mixture is exceptionally useful to keep handy and can be applied to any part of the body which is experiencing pain.

You will need to place all the ingredients into a large dark colored glass bottle. Add eight drops of Bay leaf, twelve of Helichrysum Italicum, eight of clove bud and twelve of Roman Chamomile. You will also need twelve drops of ginger, twelve of Rosemary and twelve of Lavender. Next, add four tablespoons of jojoba oil, four teaspoons of castor oil, four teaspoons of St. John's Wort oil, and two teaspoons of Calendula oil. Once all the ingredients are thoroughly mixed inside the bottle you must leave it to sit for twenty four hours. It can then be applied to any painful area as and when required.

Chapter 2 – 8 Dedicated uses for Essential Oils as Pain relief

Essential oils are generally placed on the skin and not consumed as they have powerful affects and would be highly unstable. This is not to say that a few drops of oil cannot be consumed as part of a recipe. However, most pain relief is provided faster and more effectively by applying it directly to the painful area of your body. Sometimes you will need a recipe which is designed for a specific type of pain rather than a general pain relief or prevention of muscle aches.

1. *Nerve pain*

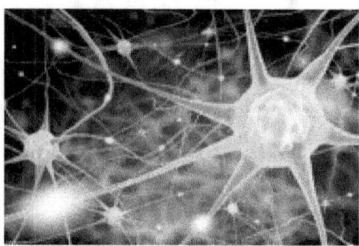

This can be one of the most difficult pains to deal with as it is unrelenting. As well as being extremely painful it can make your body tingle and can even restrict your ability to complete everyday tasks. Possibly the best reason to use the following recipe is that, once made you can apply it to the affected area as many times as you like during the course of the day.

You will need to mix it in a bottle or other suitable container which will allow you to store it and easily use a little at a time. Mix eighteen drops of lavender oil with thirty drops of Chamomile, twenty two of Majoram and another twenty two of Helichrysum. Once you have mixed these oils thoroughly add two hundred milliliters of your chosen base oil; sweet almond oil is always a good option. Mix again and then leave, out of direct sunlight, for twenty four hours before applying as needed.

2. Foot Pain

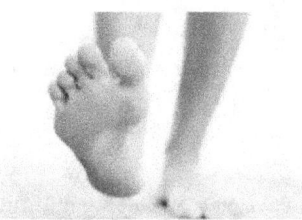

Your feet take a constant pounding. Every day they are placed inside socks and shoes, often squished more than they should be. Most people spend hours on their feet everyday; even if they have a sitting down job! Once you start exercising as well the pressures on your feet can quickly multiple and leave you need a little care and assistance.

It is important to note that this recipe is designed to reduce pain in your feet; it does not prevent you from seeking professional assistance to resolve any foot issue.

Mix eight drops of Arnica oil with eight drops of Chamomile and six drops of Rosemary. You will also need two tablespoons of base oil. Once all the ingredients have been mixed you can massage them into your feet to provide almost instant relief from pain.

It is important to note that Arnica simulates blood flow and should never be used on an open wound; this will encourage blood to flow out of the wound not healing. The Chamomile and Rosemary both provide effective anti-inflammatory treatment alongside the pain relief.

3. Back pain

This is one pain that affects the majority of people at some point in their lives. The reason for this is simply that the stresses and strains of modern life weaken your immune system and often physical strength. One of the most common places to start feeling these stresses is your lower back; part of the structure which is key to your core strength.

One of the simplest recipes is to mix twenty drops of Ginger, Lavender and Eucalyptus with four tablespoons of sweet almond oil. You can also add in twenty drops of rosemary to improve the anti-inflammatory effects of this potent mixture.

The heat of the ginger compliments the coolness of the Eucalyptus to create a soothing and relaxing experience. Ideally you or a friend should massage the mixture into your skin; if this is not possible then leaving the mixture on your skin will help it to take effect.

4. Your Knees

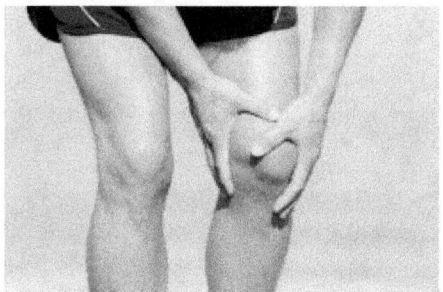

The knees take a surprising amount of stress through the course of your life. Constant flexing, impact sports and kneeling will cause wear and this will often cause pain in your knees as you age. Fortunately the following recipe can be put directly onto your knees and even used on your hips to alleviate the pain.

You will need thirty six drops of lavender oil, twenty four drops of Bergamot, twenty four drops of Marjoram and twelve drops of black pepper. This needs to be combined with 150ml of your chosen base oil. As always, sweet almond oil is a good choice. The mixture should be stored in a dark glass bottle and kept out of the sunlight. It can be used as soon as you have mixed it and applied at any time of the day.

5. Arthritis

This is something that affects a huge number of people. Your joints are used hundreds and thousands of times throughout your life, unfortunately for many people the wear and tear of this normal usage damages the joint and causes it to become stiff and painful when it is moved. This can then become an issue which prevents people from getting around comfortably. In extreme cases, people are unable to straighten or bend limbs properly.

This recipe will provide immediate relief: Place 100ml of sweet almond oil in a dark glass bottle and add thirty drops of Helichrysum, ten drops of Spruce, ten drops of Peppermint and ten drops of Eucalyptus. As well as reducing pain it will reduce any inflammation in the joints; making them easier to move. The mixture should be left for twenty four hours before you use it; then simply apply it to the affected area as and when needed.

6. Arthritic Bath

An alternative or supplementary essential oils recipe to help with arthritis is the following bath oil mixture. As its name suggests, this mixture should be added to your bath whilst you are running it. You can then climb in and relax; the essential oils will ease your aches. Ideally you should spend at least fifteen minutes in the bath.

To make your mixture add 10ml of sweet almond oil to five drops of Lavender, five of Cypress and just two drops of Ginger. Once combined simply add it to the bath water and enjoy!

7. Arthritic Massage

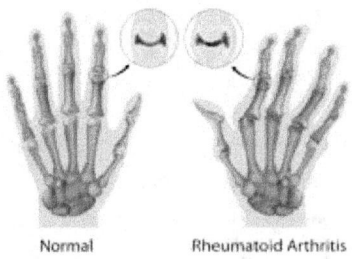

Normal   Rheumatoid Arthritis

https://userscontent2.emaze.com/images/7cd9cfe5-1d31-4268-a53f-9d44f37b5910/3366bbde-ef79-46c3-acd7-007514f7a249.jpg

Massage is still one of the best ways to get these essential oils into your system where they can have the most effect on any damaged joints and muscles thereby reducing or eliminating the pain.

This particular recipe uses several strong oils and you may find that you prefer the same oils in a slightly weaker dose. There is no reason you cannot adjust the recipe to fit your particular tastes or preferences. The following mixture is designed to provide pain relief, reduce inflammation and improve the blood flow around your body.

You will need two hundred milliliters of sweet almond oil, sixty drops of Helichrysum, sixty drops of Sweet Birch, sixty drops of Peppermint and twenty of Ginger. Mix them thoroughly and they will be ready to use instantly. It is important to just dab a little onto the specific area at first to ensure you are comfortable with the results.

8. Hand pain

Hand pain is also often associated with arthritis although there are many other reasons why your hands may ache. Regardless of what has caused the ache you will be able to find relief by simply mixing ten drops of black pepper oil with ten of Ginger and fifty milliliters of sweet almond oil. This can then be rubbed into your hands for almost immediate relief.

It is possible to add ten drops of Peppermint to the mix; however, this can leave your hands feeling tingly and this is not something that everyone enjoys. The choice is yours...

Chapter 3 – 8 More Pain Relieving Recipes

There are a vast number of recipes available for effective pain relief. The best way of deciding which one is suitable for your needs is to test as many as possible by making small doses of the mixtures. Once you are happy the bigger you can make your mixture providing you keep all the ingredients in proportion to each other. These recipes can be stored for long periods of time if necessary making it highly unlikely that you will waste any of your mixture.

The following eight recipes can help to ensure your aches and pains disappear quickly, leaving you free to get on with your life.

1. *Sore Muscle Mixture*

This is an alternative to the one already provided in chapter one and is also extremely effective. The slightly different mix works to heat your muscles, helping them to relax. It is designed to be used after you have completed a heavy exercise routine although it will work on sore muscles regardless of the reason for them.

You will need to mix four drops of Ginger with eight drops of Cinnamon, six drops of Chamomile and six of Cajuput. Add the mixture to thirty milliliters of sweet almond oil and it is ready to use straight away. Work it into any of the muscles which are aching and leave it to start having its magical effects.

2. Headaches

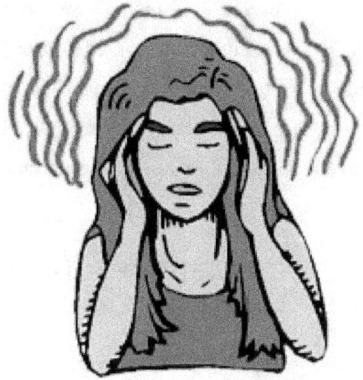

Headaches are one thing that almost everyone on the planet has suffered from at some point. They are exceptionally annoying as you are suddenly unable to do anything. Fortunately you can make a salve which you can use anytime you feel a headache coming on for remarkably quick and effective pain relief.

You will need to fill a saucepan with hot tap water and then place a bowl in this hot water; the water should not get into the bowl. Next place half a cup of coconut oil into the bowl, the heat of the hot water should melt the oil fairly quickly. You will then be able to add twenty drops of Eucalyptus, twenty of peppermint and twenty of lavender. Stir it thoroughly before pouring it into a suitable container. It should be left to cool at room temperature and then placed in the fridge for one hour before using. It is best to keep this salve in the fridge to ensure it does not liquefy. You can then apply the salve to your forehead, or your temples to obtain effective headache relief.

3. Sprain Relief

It can be very easy to sprain a joint in your body. The ankle is one of the most common partly because it is used the most and easily susceptible to a bad landing or a trip. Once you have sprained yourself you will note the area swells, bruising is common and you may have difficulty using the affected joint; which can compromise your mobility. This type of injury can take a while to heal, especially if you continue to try and use it.

The following recipe is designed to provide pain relief for your sprain and to help reduce the inflammation; in turn speeding up the healing process.

You will need to warm four teaspoons of olive oil in a small bowl. Do not boil! Once it is warm you can add twenty drops of Peppermint and twenty of Lavender. You can then apply it directly to your sprain area; whilst it is still warm. Any which is not used can be saved for another time and gently reheated. It can be used cold although it will take slightly longer to provide relief; simply because the oils will be warmed by the temperature of the skin before they soak in effectively.

4. Pain Relieving Balm

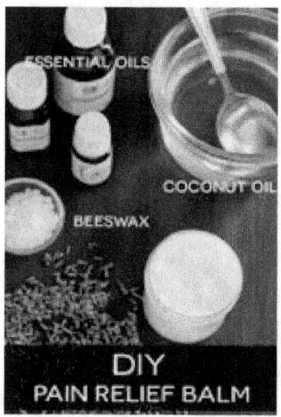

This mixture is designed to relieve pain but also to give you a boost as it has enough of a zing to make any area of your body feel revitalized.

Start by bringing a half full pan of water to the boil and then place your bowl in the water; ensuring the water does not go in the bowl. You can now place one ounce of Grapeseed oil with half an ounce of castor oil and three quarters of an ounce of beeswax into the bowl. This will gradually melt but will take a few minutes. You can stir if you wish but it is not essential.

Then add thirty drops of Peppermint, fifteen of Ginger, fifteen of Cinnamon, ten of Thyme, seven of Rosemary, ten of Clove, twenty of Frankincense, eight of Camphor, ten of Eucalyptus and fifteen of tea tree. Mix thoroughly and pour into a jar. You will need to leave it to cool before using it. You can reduce the heat of it by reducing the cinnamon content or the coolness by adjusting the Eucalyptus.

The balm can be rubbed into any part of your body where you are experiencing sore muscles. It is best to wash your hands after using the balm.

5. Slipped Disc Massage Mix

A slipped disc is extremely painful. It is often the cause of sciatica and can result in intense pain in the area of the disc as it puts pressure on your spinal column and the main nerves travelling through your body. It is essential to have any suspected slipped disc checked and treated by a medical professional.

However, whilst you are waiting to be seen and helped, the following mixture can assist in relieving the pain. It is important to note that this type of injury should be treated with ice for the first two or three days to help keep swelling to a minimum. Only after this time period can you apply the following:

Mix twenty drops of Rosemary and twenty of Peppermint with ten of Ginger and ten of Eucalyptus. All the oils need to be absorbed into a base oil; such as sweet almond or coconut. You can then dab it onto the affected disc as you need throughout the day.

6. All Over Muscle Ache

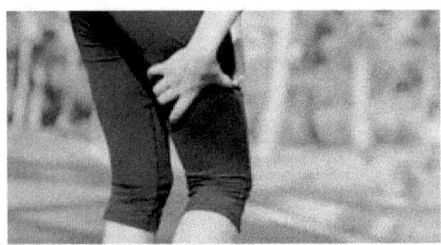

This mixture can be used on any part of your body and will provide effective, quick relief of your muscular related pain. You will need a dark colored glass bottle to mix and store the ingredients in. Simply place half a cup of olive oil in the bottle with twenty drops of black pepper, twenty four of Coriander, twelve of White grapefruit and four or five of Ginger. Once the ingredients are mixed thoroughly you can leave it to sit for two hours before massaging into the injured area after a warm bath.

7. Relieve Tension

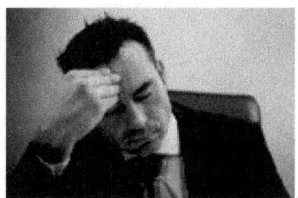

Tension is a form of stress which can quickly build up to cause issues within your body. In fact, tension can cause physical pain as well as worry and an inability to complete tasks properly. Fortunately, there are some essential oils which help to combat against this. Simply mix two tablespoons of sweet almond oil with ten drops of Melaleuca oil and ten of Lavender. Once you have mixed completely the oils can be applied to your forehead and temples; this is the most effective way of relieving tension and can also work on headaches. Coincidentally, headaches are often a result of tension in the body.

8. Headache relief

As this is one of the most infuriating and often difficult to deal with pains it is worth having more than one approach to assist you in dealing with those moments when you feel like your head will implode.

If you mix two tablespoons of base oil, such as coconut or sweet almond with five drops of each of the following oils, you will create a blend which is effective at dealing with headaches and many other pains across your body. The oils are peppermint, Eucalyptus, Rosemary; Ginger, lavender, Cinnamon, Chamomile and lemongrass.

Once mixed it can be applied immediately or stored for use at any point in the future.

Conclusion

Essential oils work differently for everyone. In fact, a recipe that some will swear by can have little effect on a best friend. This is just the way most things work and is why it is essential to make small batches of any of these recipes to allow you to test them before you commit to making and storing your own essential oil treatment.

It is also possible to simply place a few drops of the right essential oil into a bowl of hot water and then breathe in the fumes. This can be an exceptionally efficient way of removing the congestion associated with colds and flu.

Perhaps one of the best things about essential oils is the huge variety of them which are available and the range of products which can be created with them. Each of the recipes described in this book will provide effective pain relief. They are also fairly basic recipes. This provides you with the opportunity to adjust each recipe according to your own tastes and needs. This is particularly relevant if you find that one does not have the desired effect. You can increase the hotter or cooler oils or simply substitute one for another to help create something that does exactly what you want it to.

It is essential to note that essential or aromatic oils are volatile. This means you should always use separate equipment when preparing them and not your standard cooking utensils. You should also wear gloves to protect your hands from any potential burns which may be caused by splashing the concentrated oil.

You will note every one of these recipes significantly dilutes the oils to create the desired effect; this is a health precaution. Even the fumes can be dangerous if breathed in concentrated for extensive periods of time.

Creating your own pain relief remedies from completely natural resources is going to save you a significant amount of funds. It is also going to make you feel very satisfied as you have managed to create pain relief without causing any harm to the environment. In fact, you are following in the footsteps of our ancestors and learning to use what is readily available from nature. Even the commercial pain relief drugs use plant extracts along with a variety of man-made substances to provide effective pain relief. Once you have tried a few of these recipes you will realize that it is possible to achieve just as effective a pain relief but without the synthetic chemicals which could be doing as much harm as good to your body.

The majority of these recipes can be prepared and stored now. Providing they are clearly labeled you will simply be able to grab what you need when you feel the pain start. This will ensure you have fast and effective relief, when you need it. With just a few small bottles of essential oils in your cupboard you will also be able to continue creating effective pain relief for a significant amount of time. However, it is important to note that if you are experiencing pain long term, stopping the pain is not enough; you should have yourself checked by a medical professional.

FREE Bonus Reminder

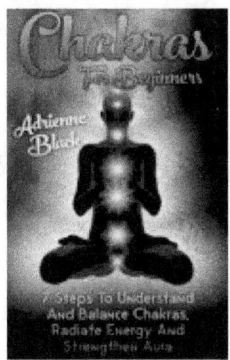

If you have not grabbed it yet, please go ahead and download your special bonus E book *"Chakras for Beginners. 7 Steps To Understand And Balance Chakras, Radiate Energy, And Strengthen Aura"*.

Simply Click the Button Below

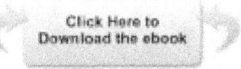

OR Go to This Page

http://lifehacksworld.com/free

BONUS #2: More Free & Discounted Books & Products

Do you want to receive more Free/Discounted Books or Products?

We have a mailing list where we send out our new Books or Products when they go free or with a discount on Amazon. Click on the link below to sign up for Free & Discount Book & Product Promotions.

=> Sign Up for Free & Discount Book & Product Promotions <=

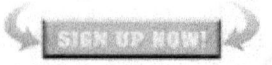

OR Go to this URL

http://zbit.ly/1WBb1Ek

www.ingramcontent.com/pod-product-compliance
Lightning Source LLC
Chambersburg PA
CBHW071323280526
45788CB00004B/1998